MODERN BREATHING,
the old fashion way

MODERN BREATHING,
the old fashion way

A modern, common usage American English
translation of Yogi Ramacharaka's classic, *The Hindu-
Yogi Science of Breathing*.

Re-organized, Translated and Edited by
Lewis A. Clarke

Introductory Note

This new text is intended for all those modern mouth breathers, like me, who are too busy chasing life and being chased by it, to stop and take a deep breath. I have consolidated all the exercises into a brief linear format so you can start adjusting your breathing mechanics immediately.

There will be disagreement with my leaving some of the explanations and reasoning behind the exercises, their need in our modern life and their more universality implications out of this text. At this point in time I feel that your breathing health is more important. Discover what works for you. Feel better. Then explore more.

LAC

CONTENTS

The Four Methods of Respiration

The Complete Breath

Three Important Additional Methods

Seven Developmental Exercises

Seven Minor Exercises

Rhythmic Breathing

MODERN BREATHING,
the old fashion way

The Four Methods of Respiration

The mechanics of respiration are "simple." The elastic movements of the lungs and the muscular contractions and expansions of the sides and bottom of the thoracic cavity expand the lungs and air is pulled in and expelled. Without these muscular contractions and expansions respiration would not happen. The proper control of these muscles will result in your ability to attain the maximum degree of lung expansion and the greatest amount of oxygen pulled into your system.

There are four general methods of respiration:

(1) High Breathing.
(2) Mid Breathing.
(3) Low Breathing.
(4) Complete Breathing.

A general description of the four methods follows with a comprehensive look at the Complete Breath afterwards.

(1) HIGH BREATHING

(Shallow breathing, or chest breathing or upper lobar breathing, or clavicular breathing, or clavicle breathing) like a mouth breather

Breathing this way you elevate your ribs and raise the collarbone and shoulders, at the same time drawing in the abdomen and pushing its contents up against the diaphragm, which in turn is raised.

The upper part of the chest and lungs, which is the smallest, is used, and consequently a minimum amount of air enters the lungs. In addition to this, the diaphragm being raised, there can be no expansion in that direction.

High Breathing is probably the worst form of breathing known to man and requires the greatest expenditure of energy with the smallest amount of benefit. It is a lose-lose process.

(2) MID BREATHING

(Intercostal breathing) like an athlete catching their breath

In Mid-Breathing the diaphragm is pushed upward, and the abdomen drawn in. The ribs are raised somewhat, and the chest is partially expanded filling the top third of the lungs, as in clavicular breathing, and then continuing down into the middle part of the lungs.

(3) LOW BREATHING

(Abdominal Breathing, Belly Breathing,
Diaphragmatic Breathing) like a sleeping baby

In Low Breathing, the diaphragm drives the lungs
action and more air is inhaled in a more relaxed action.
But Low Breathing only fills the lower and middle area
of the lungs.

(4) COMPLETE BREATH

The Complete Breath is a combination of Low, Mid and High Breaths but it **is not** three distinct movements. It is a continuous, uniform, inhalation incorporating the beneficial points of High Breathing, Mid Breathing and Low Breathing. With the Complete Breath your chest cavity is increased to its normal limits in all directions.

The muscles controlling the ribs expand, increasing the space for the lungs to expand. The lower ribs are drawn downward by the diaphragm and the upper ribs are lifted up and out outward.

The Complete Breath Exercise

You may find it quite helpful to practice in front of a mirror.

(1) Stand or sit erect. Inhale steadily through your nostrils filling the lower part of your lungs. (This is accomplished by the descending your diaphragm.) Continuing to inhale, fill the middle part of the lungs by pushing out your lower ribs, breast-bone and chest. Extend your upper chest outward and fill your upper lungs. During this last motion your lower abdomen will be slightly drawn in.) lungs.

The Complete Breath is a combination of Low, Mid and High Breaths but it **is not** three distinct movements. It is a continuous, uniform, inhalation. Practice.

(2) Retain the breath a few seconds.

(3) Exhale quite slowly. Keep Your chest in a firm position, your stomach sucked in a little, raising the diaphragm upward slowly as the air leaves your lungs.

(4) Relax.

It is considered good practice to lift your shoulders slightly as you finish your inhalation. This raises your collarbone allowing fresh air to fill the small upper lobe of your right lung.

9

Three Important Additional Methods

CLEANSING BREATH

This Cleansing Breath ventilates and cleanses the lungs, stimulates the cells and gives a general tone to the respiratory organs, and is conducive to their general healthy condition. Besides this effect, it is found to greatly refresh the entire system.

(1) Inhale a complete breath.
(2) Retain the air a few seconds.
(3) Pucker up the lips as if for a whistle (but do not swell out the cheeks), then exhale a little air through the opening, with considerable vigor. Stop for a moment, retaining the air, and then exhale a little more air.
(4) Repeat until the air is completely exhaled.

Remember that considerable vigor is to be used in exhaling the air through the opening in the lips.

This breath will be found quite refreshing when you are tired. It should be practiced until it can be performed naturally and easily, as it is used to finish up a number of other exercises given in this book. It should be thoroughly understood.

VITALIZING BREATH

This exercise brings a stimulating pressure to bear on important nerve centers, which in turn stimulate and energize the entire nervous system, and send an increased flow of nerve force to all parts of the body.

(1) Stand erect.

(2) Inhale a Complete Breath.

(3) Extend your arms out in front of you, letting them be somewhat limp and relaxed, with only sufficient nerve force to hold them out.

(4) Slowly draw your hands back toward your shoulders, gradually contracting your hands into a fist so that when they reach the shoulders the fists will be tightly clenched.

(5) Keeping the muscles tense, push the fists slowly out, and then draw them back rapidly (still tense) several times.

(6) Exhale vigorously through the mouth.

(7) Practice the Cleansing Breath.

The efficiency of this exercise depends greatly upon the speed of the drawing back of the fists, and the tension of the muscles, and, of course, upon the full lungs.

13

VOCAL BREATH

The exercise given below is to be used only as an occasional exercise, and not as a regular form of breathing.

(1) Inhale a Complete Breath very slowly, but steadily, through the nostrils, taking as much time as possible in the inhalation.

(2) Retain for a few seconds.

(3) Expel the air vigorously in one great breath, through the wide opened mouth.

(4) Rest the lungs by the Cleansing Breath.

The Exercises

Seven Developmental Exercises

The following seven exercises are for developing the lungs, muscles, ligaments, air cells, etc. They are simple but effective. Do not allow their simplicity to make you lose interest.

(1) THE RETAINED BREATH

This is a very important exercise which helps strengthen and develop the respiratory muscles as well as the lungs. Its frequent practice will help to expand the chest. The occasional holding of your breath tends to purify the air which has remained in the lungs from former inhalations, and to more fully oxygenate the blood. The retained breath gathers up waste matter, and when expelled, cleanses the lungs.

At first you may only be able to retain the breath for a short time, but with a little practice you will improve. Time yourself with a watch if you wish to note your progress.

Pay attention to this exercise. It has great merit.

(1) Stand erect.
(2) Inhale a Complete Breath.
(3) Retain the air as long as you can comfortably.
(4) Exhale vigorously through your mouth.
(5) Practice the Cleansing Breath.

(2) LUNG CELL STIMULATION BREATH

This exercise is designed to stimulate the air cells in the lungs. It is very bracing and stimulating to the whole body. Do not not overdo it. You may experience a slight dizziness the first few times you try it. If so, discontinue the exercise for a while, trials, walk around a little.

(1) Stand erect, with hands at sides.
(2) Breathe in very slowly and gradually.
(3) While inhaling, gently tap the chest with the finger tips, constantly changing position.
(4) When the lungs are filled, retain the breath and pat the chest with the palms of the hands.
(5) Practice the Cleansing Breath.

(3) RIB STRETCHING BREATH

In proper breathing, the ribs play an important part, and it is well to occasionally give them a little special exercise in order to preserve their elasticity. Standing or sitting in unnatural positions is apt to render the ribs more or less stiff and inelastic. This exercise will do much to overcome that.

(1) Stand erect.

(2) Place your hands on each side of the body, as high up under the armpits as convenient, the thumbs reaching toward the back, the palms on the side of the chest and the fingers to the front over the breast.

(3) Inhale a Complete Breath.

(4) Retain the air for a short time.

(5) Then gently squeeze the sides, at the same time slowly exhaling.

(6) Practice the cleansing breath.

Use moderation in this exercise and do not overdo it.

(4) CHEST EXPANSION BREATH

In modern styles of work the chest is quite apt to be contracted from bending over or slumping. This exercise is very good for restoring your natural conditions and gaining chest expansion.

(1) Stand erect.
(2) Inhale a Complete Breath.
(3) Retain the air.
(4) Extend both arms forward and bring the two clenched fists together on a level with the shoulder.
(5) Swing back the fists vigorously until the arms stand out straight sideways from the shoulders.
(6) Then bring back to Position 4, and swing to Position 5. Repeat several times.
(7) Exhale vigorously through the opened mouth.
(8) Practice the Cleansing Breath.

Use moderation and do not overdo this exercise.

(5) WALKING EXERCISE BREATH

(1) Walk with head up, chin drawn slightly in, shoulders back, and with measured tread.

(2) Inhale a Complete Breath, counting (mentally) 1, 2, 3,4, 5, 6, 7, 8, one count to each step, making the inhalation extend over the eight counts.

(3) Exhale slowly through the nostrils, counting as before, 1, 2, 3, 4, 5, 6, 7, 8, one count to a step.

(4) Rest between breaths, continuing walking and counting, 1, 2, 3, 4, 5, 8, 7, 8, one count to a step.

(5) Repeat until you begin to feel tired. Then rest for awhile, and resume at your leisure. Repeat several times a day.

You can vary this exercise by retaining the breath during a 1, 2, 3, 4, count, and then exhaling in an eight-step count. Practice whichever plan is more comfortable for you.

(6) MORNING EXERCISE BREATH

(1) Stand erect in a military attitude, head up, eyes front, shoulders back, knees stiff, hands at sides.

(2) Raise up slowly on your toes, inhaling a Complete Breath, steadily and slowly.

(3) Retain the breath for a few seconds, maintaining the raised position.

(4) Slowly return to the lower position while slowly exhaling through your nostrils.

(5) Practice Cleansing Breath.

(6) Repeat several times, varying by using right leg alone, then left leg alone.

(7) STIMULATING CIRCULATION BREATH

(1) Stand erect.

(2) Inhale a Complete Breath and retain.

(3) Bend forward slightly and grasp a stick or cane steadily and firmly. Gradually exert your entire strength upon your grasp.

(4) Relax your grasp, return to first position, and slowly exhale.

(5) Repeat several times.

(6) Finish with the Cleansing Breath.

This exercise may be performed without the use of a stick or cane, by grasping an imaginary cane, using the will to exert the pressure.

The exercise stimulates circulation by driving the arterial blood to the extremities and drawing back the depleted blood to the heart and lungs so that it may be re-oxygenated. It is well to practice this exercise, occasionally with the regular Complete Breathing exercise.

Seven Minor Exercises

This chapter is composed of seven exercises, bearing no special names. Each is distinct and separate from the others and have a different purpose in view. You may find one or more of these exercises to be just what you need. Do not pass them by because they are marked "minor." Try them and decide for yourself.

EXERCISE I

(1) Stand erect with hands at your sides.

(2) Inhale a Complete Breath.

(3) Raise your arms slowly, keeping them rigid until your hands touch over your head.

(4) Retain your breath a few minutes with your hands over head.

(5) Lower your hands slowly to your sides, exhaling slowly.

(6) Practice the Cleansing Breath.

EXERCISE II

(1) Stand erect, with arms straight in front of you.

(2) Inhale a Complete Breath and retain.

(3) Swing arms back as far as they will go; then back to the front; repeating several times, retaining your breath.

(4) Exhale vigorously through your mouth.

(5) Practice the Cleansing Breath.

EXERCISE III

(1) Stand erect with your arms straight out in front of you,

(2) Inhale a Complete Breath.

(3) Swing your arms around in a circle, backward, a few times. Then reverse the rotation while retaining your breath.

(4) Exhale the breath vigorously through the mouth.

(5) Practice the Cleansing Breath.

EXERCISE IV

(1) Lie on the floor face down with your palms flat upon the floor by your sides.

(2) Inhale a Complete Breath and retain.

3) Stiffen your body and raise yourself up by the strength of your arms until you rest on your hands and toes

(4) Then lower yourself to original position. Repeat several times.

(5) Exhale vigorously through your mouth.

(6) Practice the Cleansing Breath.

EXERCISE V

(1) Stand erect with your palms against the wall.

(2) Inhale a Complete Breath and retain.

(3) Resting your weight on your hands lower your chest to the wall,.

(4) Keeping your body stiff, raise yourself back with your arm muscles alone,.

(5) Exhale vigorously through the mouth.

(6) Practice the Cleansing Breath.

EXERCISE VI

(1) Stand erect with arms "akimbo," that is, with hands resting around the waist and elbows standing out.

(2) Inhale a Complete Breath and retain.

(3) Keep your legs and hips stiff and bend well forward, as if bowing, at the same time exhaling slowly.

(4) Return to the first position and take another Complete Breath.

(5) Then bend backward, exhaling slowly.

(6) Return to first position and take a Complete Breath.

(7) Then bend sideways, exhaling slowly. (Vary by bending to right and then to left.)

(8) Practice a Cleansing Breath.

EXERCISE VII

(1) Stand erect, or sit erect, with straight spinal column.

(2) Inhale a Complete Breath, but instead of inhaling in a continuous steady stream, take a series of short, quick "sniffs," as if you were smelling aromatic salts or ammonia and did not wish to get too strong a "whiff." Do not exhale any of these little breaths, but add one to the other until the entire lung space Is filled.

(3) Retain for a few seconds.

(4) Exhale through the nostrils in a long, restful, sighing breath.

(5) Practice a Cleansing Breath.

Rhythmic Breathing

The rule for rhythmic breathing is that the units of inhalation and exhalation should be the same, while the units for retention and between breaths should be one-half the number of those of inhalation and exhalation.

Your heart beat is the proper rhythmic standard for your rhythmic breathing. Ascertain your normal heart beat by placing your fingers over your pulse, and then count: "1, 2, 3, 4, 5, 6; 1, 2, 3, 4, 5, 6," etc., until the rhythm becomes firmly fixed in your mind. A little practice will fix the rhythm, so that you will be able to easily reproduce it. The beginner usually inhales in about six pulse units, but you will be able to greatly increase this by practice.

RHYTHMIC BREATH

(1) Sit erect, in an easy posture, hold your chest, neck and head as nearly in a straight line as possible, with shoulders slightly thrown back, hands resting easily in your lap.

2) Slowly inhale a Complete Breath, counting six pulse units.

(3) Retain, counting three pulse units.

(4) Exhale slowly through the nostrils, counting six pulse units.

(5) Count three pulse beats, then repeat the process.

(6) You can repeat a number of times, but avoid fatiguing yourself at the start.

(7) When you are ready to close the exercise, practice the cleansing breath, which will rest you and cleanse your lungs.

After a little practice you will be able to increase the duration of the inhalations and exhalations, up to about fifteen pulse units. In this increase, remember that the units for retention and between breaths is one-half the units for inhalation and exhalation.

Do not overdo yourself. Pay attention to acquiring the "rhythm." It is more important than the length of the breath.

41